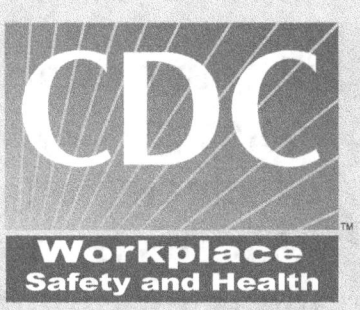

Evaluation of Chemical Hazards and Noise Exposures at a Drum Refurbishing Plant – Indiana

Kenneth W. Fent, PhD
Elena Page, MD, MPH
Scott E. Brueck, MS, CIH

Health Hazard Evaluation Report
HETA 2010-0031-3130
June 2011

DEPARTMENT OF HEALTH AND HUMAN SERVICES
Centers for Disease Control and Prevention

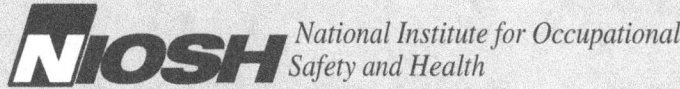

National Institute for Occupational
Safety and Health

The employer shall post a copy of this report for a period of 30 calendar days at or near the workplace(s) of affected employees. The employer shall take steps to insure that the posted determinations are not altered, defaced, or covered by other material during such period. [37 FR 23640, November 7, 1972, as amended at 45 FR 2653, January 14, 1980].

CONTENTS

REPORT

Abbreviations ii

Highlights of the NIOSH Health Hazard Evaluation iii

Summary v

Introduction 1

Assessment 3

Results 5

Discussion 11

Conclusions 14

Recommendations..14

References..18

APPENDIX A:

Methods...19

APPENDIX B:

Occupational Exposure Limits and Health Effects......................21

ACKNOWLEDGMENTS

Acknowledgments and Availability of Report...............................27

ABBREVIATIONS

ACGIH®	American Conference of Governmental Industrial Hygienists
AL	Action level
CFR	Code of Federal Regulations
dB	Decibels
dBA	Decibels, A-weighted
HHE	Health hazard evaluation
HTL	Hearing threshold level
Hz	Hertz
MDC	Minimum detectable concentration
mg	Milligrams
mg/m^3	Milligrams per cubic meter
MQC	Minimum quantifiable concentration
MSDS	Material safety data sheet
NAICS	North American Industry Classification System
ND	Not detected
NIOSH	National Institute for Occupational Safety and Health
OEL	Occupational exposure limit
OSHA	Occupational Safety and Health Administration
PBZ	Personal breathing zone
PEL	Permissible exposure limit
PPE	Personal protective equipment
PVC	Polyvinyl chloride
REL	Recommended exposure limit
SLM	Sound level meter
STS	Standard threshold shift
STEL	Short-term exposure limit
TLV®	Threshold limit value
TTS	Temporary threshold shift
TWA	Time-weighted average
VOC	Volatile organic compound
WEEL™	Workplace environmental exposure level

HIGHLIGHTS OF THE NIOSH HEALTH HAZARD EVALUATION

The National Institute for Occupational Safety and Health (NIOSH) received a confidential employee request for a health hazard evaluation at a drum refurbishing plant in Indiana. The requestors reported respiratory irritation, chemical burns, and headaches from exposure to chemicals in the drums. Employees were also concerned about exposure to noise.

What NIOSH Did

- We evaluated the plant in February 2010 and again in March 2010.

- We observed the work being done at the plant. We also asked employees about their work and medical history and if they had any symptoms or health concerns related to their work.

- We measured aromatic hydrocarbons and sodium hydroxide levels in the air.

- We measured noise exposures.

What NIOSH Found

- Most employees said they had no symptoms related to their work. Some employees did, however, report symptoms that were consistent with airborne exposure to solvents.

- We measured trimethyl benzene levels above occupational exposure limits (OELs) in the tote wash department. All other air sampling results were below OELs.

- There was potential for skin exposure to solvents throughout the plant.

- All noise exposures were above the NIOSH recommended exposure limit and the Occupational Safety and Health Administration (OSHA) Action Level of 85 A-weighted decibels (dBA).

- Pressure washing of drums and totes resulted in the highest noise levels in the plant. Some of these noise exposures exceeded 100 dBA.

- The plant had no health and safety committee.

What Managers Can Do

- Replace Aromatic 100 with a less hazardous solvent for cleaning the outside of the totes and drums.

- Add local exhaust ventilation where drums and totes are emptied and cleaned.

- Install an exhaust hood over drums used to collect residual waste emptied from the totes.

- Partially enclose or install a barrier where drums and totes are pressure washed. This will help reduce noise levels in nearby work areas.

- Require employees to use both earplugs and earmuffs in areas where noise exposures are greater than 100 decibels (dB). Earplugs and earmuffs should be provided to employees.

- Follow Indiana OSHA's recommendation to separate the cleaning of drums and totes according to the types of chemicals they contain. This separation will help prevent chemical reactions that could produce other hazardous chemicals.

- Develop a list of required personal protective equipment (PPE) for each job task. This list should be based on a review of hazards.

- Retrain employees how to properly wear and maintain the PPE.

- Start a health and safety committee that meets regularly to discuss concerns at the plant. This committee should have both employee and management representation.

What Employees Can Do

- Wear and maintain all your PPE correctly.

- Wear earplugs and earmuffs in work areas where noise exposures are above 100 dB.

- Participate in the health and safety committee.

- Report symptoms related to work to your supervisor or the plant safety manager.

SUMMARY

NIOSH investigators evaluated a drum refurbishing plant in Indiana because of reports of noise, respiratory irritation, chemical burns, and headaches. Although the symptoms reported were consistent with exposures to solvents, most airborne exposures to aromatic hydrocarbons were below OELs. However, one employee was overexposed to trimethyl benzene. Employees throughout the plant had the potential for dermal exposure to solvents and other chemicals. All personal noise exposure measurements exceeded NIOSH and OSHA OELs for an 8-hour workday.

In December 2009 NIOSH received a confidential employee request for an HHE at a drum refurbishing plant in Indiana. The requestors reported respiratory irritation, chemical burns, and headaches from exposure to chemicals present in the drums. They were also concerned about noise exposure. In response to this HHE request, we conducted evaluations on February 2, 2010, and March 22–23, 2010.

We interviewed employees during our first visit. We asked them about their job history, personal medical history, and if they had any symptoms or health concerns related to their work. We reviewed the OSHA 300 Logs of Work-related Injuries and Illnesses for the years 2006 to 2009 and emergency room records for one employee who reported seeking care after exposure to chemicals on the job.

During our second visit, we conducted PBZ sampling for VOCs, aromatic hydrocarbons, and sodium hydroxide. We measured full-shift TWA personal noise exposures. We measured sound levels and conducted one-third octave band frequency analysis from 12.5 Hz to 20,000 Hz throughout production areas of the plant.

Of the 21 employees we interviewed, only four reported symptoms they believed were related to work. Two of these employees reported headaches, two reported eye irritation, one reported dizziness, and one reported sinus infections. The OSHA Logs documented one employee with an STS in an audiogram in 2009, one employee with burning eyes in 2007, and four employees with chemical burns in 2006. One employee sought emergency room care for cough and chest pain after breathing in chemicals at work and was treated with a bronchodilator and released with an inhaler to use for shortness of breath.

All aromatic hydrocarbon exposures were below applicable OELs except one PBZ concentration of trimethyl benzene (150 mg/m^3) that exceeded the NIOSH REL and ACGIH TLV of 125 mg/m^3. This PBZ sample was from a tote wash department employee who wiped the exterior of the totes with Aromatic 100. No sodium hydroxide was detected (MDC 0.04 mg/m^3) in any of the samples.

PVC gloves with a cotton lining were provided to the employees but are not protective against Aromatic 100. Half-mask N95 filtering facepiece respirators were available to employees for voluntary use. However, we observed employees who were

SUMMARY
(CONTINUED)

improperly wearing and maintaining these respirators. Some employees believed that these respirators protected them against vapors and gases; however, these respirators are only effective against particles.

All personal noise exposure measurements exceeded the NIOSH REL and the OSHA AL of 85 dBA for an 8-hour work shift. Noise exposures for employees loading drums, wiping exteriors of drums with Dissolve II, pressure washing drums and totes, emptying and vacuuming drums, and removing labels from totes all exceeded the OSHA PEL of 90 dBA. The drum and tote pressure washers had TWA noise exposures above 100 dBA.

We recommended substituting Aromatic 100 with a less hazardous solvent for cleaning the outside of the totes and drums and adding local exhaust ventilation where drums and totes are being emptied and cleaned. Installation of an exhaust hood over drums used to collect residual waste emptied from the totes would remove any potentially hazardous chemicals that evaporate from the drums. We also recommended partially enclosing or installing barrier walls in the noisiest areas of the plant to reduce noise levels in the adjacent work areas. The company should require dual hearing protection (earplugs and earmuffs) for the employees who pressure wash drums and totes until TWA noise exposures are reduced to below 100 dBA. We advised the company to conduct a comprehensive hazard assessment to facilitate the selection of PPE as required by OSHA [29 CFR 1910.132]. Once this assessment is complete, employees need to be retrained on how to properly wear and maintain PPE, including hearing protection, gloves, sleeve covers, and safety glasses.

Keywords: NAICS 423840 (Industrial Supplies Merchant and Wholesalers), drum refurbishing, noise, chemicals, trimethyl benzene

INTRODUCTION

In December 2009 NIOSH received a confidential employee request for an HHE at a drum refurbishing plant in Indiana. The requestors reported respiratory irritation, chemical burns, and headaches from exposure to a variety of chemicals present in the drums. They were also concerned about noise exposure. In response to this HHE request, we conducted evaluations on February 2, 2010, and March 22–23, 2010.

The plant had about 50 employees. At the time of our evaluation, they were operating one 8-hour shift per day, 3–4 days per week. The plant received 55-gallon drums and 275- or 330-gallon totes that once held various chemicals. The most common types of chemicals stored in the drums were caustics and acids. The company accepted only containers that were "Resource Conservation and Recovery Act empty," which they defined as drip-dry nonviscous material or up to 1 inch of viscous material. The totes were plastic surrounded by a supporting steel mesh; most of the drums were plastic. The plant also refurbished steel drums, but none were being cleaned during our evaluations. Drums and totes were emptied of residual chemicals, cleaned, and then either shipped to customers for reuse or recycled.

Drum Refurbishing

After being unloaded outdoors, the drums were sent to the poly wash department on a conveyor belt (Figure 1). An employee manually removed labels and loaded the drums into a machine that flushed the drums with water containing 5% sodium hydroxide. Residual chemicals in the drums were emptied into a collection tank that fed into the onsite water treatment plant. After the drums exited the flush machine, an employee placed the drums on a conveyor belt and removed remaining labels with a putty knife and Dissolve II (Aztec Corporation, Indianapolis, Indiana). Dissolve II is a gel-like substance that contains a petroleum hydrocarbon mixture and dipropylene glycol monomethyl ether. The conveyor belt then carried the drums to an employee who used pressurized water to wash the exterior of the drums. Afterwards, another employee scrubbed the drums with a sponge containing Dissolve II. From here, the drums entered an automated system for further cleaning and then for drying. After the drums exited the automated cleaning system, employees visually inspected and pressure tested the drums for leaks, then rebung the drums. In the final steps, an employee wiped the exterior of the drums with a rag containing Aromatic 100 (Univar USA Inc., Kirkland,

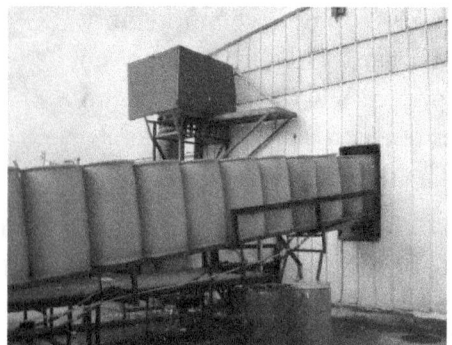

Figure 1. Plastic drums entering the drum refurbishing plant on a conveyor belt.

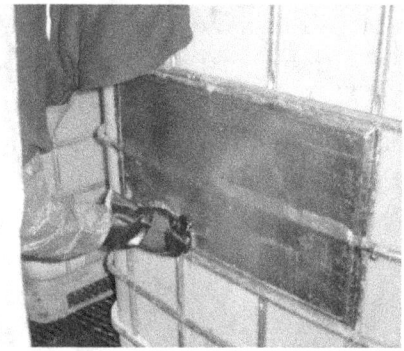

Figure 2. Employee using sponge containing Aromatic 100 to remove adhesive from the plaque of the tote.

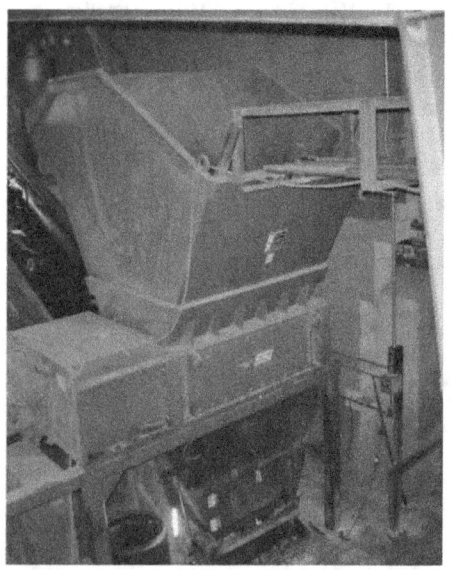

Figure 3. Grinder used for recycling plastic drums.

Washington) to remove residual markings. Aromatic 100 is a liquid that contains petroleum hydrocarbons, trimethyl benzene, xylene, and cumene. If needed, an employee touched up the drums with latex paint (ACE, Matteson, IL) using a pressurized spray gun inside a partially enclosed cross-draft ventilation booth. The paint contained 1,2-propylene glycol. The drums were stored nearby until they could be loaded onto trucks for shipping to customers.

Tote Refurbishing

After unloading, totes were carried to the tote wash department with a forklift and then machine-lifted onto a grated elevated platform. Rollers in the floor of the platform allowed employees to push the totes to the different stations. Residual chemicals in the totes were drained into open head 55-gallon drums sitting below the platform. Each week, approximately four of these drums were filled with residual chemicals for disposal. An employee removed labels from the plaque of the totes using a heater gun, putty knife, and occasionally a brush containing Dissolve II. Another employee used a sponge containing Aromatic 100 to remove adhesive and other markings on the totes (Figure 2). The totes were then automatically and repeatedly flushed with water to clean the interior. Afterwards, an employee used pressurized water to clean the exterior of the totes. After drying, the employees visually inspected and pressure tested the totes for leaks. Last, the totes were revalved, transported using a forklift, and stored or loaded onto trucks for shipment to customers.

Drum Recycling

After being unloaded, drums that had exceeded their lifespan or had leaks were sent to the regrind department on a conveyor belt. To empty the drums of residual chemicals, an employee took the drums and turned them upside down over a grated collection tank. The collection tank fed into the onsite water treatment plant. The employee then used a vacuum to remove other chemicals remaining in the drums. Afterwards, the drums were stacked next to the grinder. When enough drums were present to run the grinder, the drums were lifted on a platform to the second level of the plant. Employees then manually fed the drums into the hopper of the grinder. The grinder was a machine that shredded the drums into small pieces of plastic that were cleaned, collected, and shipped to plastic recyclers (Figure 3). The grinder typically ran once or twice per week.

Introduction (continued)

Indiana OSHA conducted an inspection at this plant between April 18, 2010, and December 20, 2010, and issued several citations. Many of these citations pertained to the mixing of incompatible chemicals. According to the *Safety Order and Notification of Penalty* from this inspection [IOSHA 2011], acids, bases, oxidizers, flammables, combustibles, other highly toxic chemicals, and suspected or confirmed carcinogens could mix together when dumped from drums into collection tanks or from totes into collection drums. The mixing of these chemicals could cause violent exothermic reactions or release hazardous decomposition products such as carbon monoxide, chlorine, ammonia, phosgene, phosphine, hydrogen, hydrogen chloride, hydrogen fluoride, hydrogen cyanide, and oxides of nitrogen and sulfur. Indiana OSHA recommended that the cleaning of drums and totes be segregated according to the type of chemicals they contain to prevent the mixing of incompatible chemicals. Other citations [IOSHA 2011] included violations of standards related to hearing conservation [29 CFR 1910.95], emergency response [29 CFR 1910.120], PPE [29 CFR 1910.133], confined spaces [29 CFR 1910.146], electrical safety [29 CFR 1910.303], and hazard communication [29 CFR 1910.1200].

Assessment

We interviewed employees during our first visit. We serially selected employees from a roster for interviews that were conducted in a private room. We asked the employees about their job history, personal medical history, and if they had symptoms or health concerns related to job exposures. We reviewed the OSHA 300 Log of Work-related Injuries and Illnesses for the years 2006 to 2009. We also reviewed emergency room records for one employee who reported seeking care after exposure to chemicals on the job.

During our second visit, we conducted PBZ sampling for VOCs, aromatic hydrocarbons, and sodium hydroxide. These samples were collected from employees who worked in the poly wash department, the tote wash department, and the regrind department over 2 days. We collected eight VOC samples from five employees performing four job tasks. These samples were collected for less than 3 hours during the 8-hour work shift. Unlike the other samples we collected, the VOC samples were qualitative in nature, which means chemicals can be identified but not their concentrations. The purpose of these samples was to determine the primary volatile constituents in the air.

ASSESSMENT
(CONTINUED)

We collected 14 aromatic hydrocarbon samples from nine employees performing eight job tasks. These samples were collected over the entire work shift (approximately 8 hours). On the basis of results of the VOC samples and the compounds listed in the MSDS for Dissolve II and Aromatic 100, we analyzed these samples for cumene, ethylbenzene, naphthalene, toluene, trimethyl benzene, xylene, and benzene. The results were averaged over the sampling period and compared to the following work-shift OELs: the NIOSH REL [NIOSH 2005], the legally enforceable OSHA PEL [NIOSH 2005], and the ACGIH TLV® [ACGIH 2010] (Table 1).

Table 1. OELs as TWA concentrations over a work shift (mg/m³)

	Cumene	Ethylbenzene	Naphthalene	Toluene	Trimethyl benzene	Xylene	Benzene
NIOSH REL	245	435	50	375	125	435	0.32
OSHA PEL	245	435	50	750	none	435	3.2
ACGIH TLV	245	435	50	75	125	435	1.6

We collected four sodium hydroxide samples from three employees performing two job tasks. These samples were collected over short time periods (~15 minutes) at processes where caustic wash (5% sodium hydroxide) was used to rinse the inside of the drums. Because sodium hydroxide was measured over ~15 minutes, STELs or ceiling limits are most applicable. The NIOSH REL and ACGIH TLV ceiling limit for sodium hydroxide are 2 mg/m³. OSHA has not promulgated a STEL or ceiling limit for sodium hydroxide. More information on the sampling methods is provided in Appendix A. More information on OELs and potential health effects for the chemicals we monitored is provided in Appendix B.

We measured work-shift TWA personal noise exposures of 26 employees using Larson Davis (Provo, Utah) Spark™ Model 705P integrating noise dosimeters. We used a Larson Davis Model 824 integrating sound level meter and real time frequency analyzer for sound level and one-third octave band frequency analysis throughout production areas of the facility. Octave band measurements were taken at frequencies from 12.5 Hz to 20,000 Hz. Noise monitoring methods are further described in Appendix A.

Employee Interviews

The 21 interviewed employees were from all areas of the plant, and all were involved in drum refurbishing. They had worked at the plant for an average of 9 years (range: 2–21 years). Seventeen reported no work-related symptoms. Two reported headache, two reported eye irritation, one reported dizziness when odors were especially strong, and one reported sinus infections since beginning work at the plant.

The OSHA 300 Logs documented one employee with a significant threshold shift in an audiogram in 2009, one employee with burning eyes in 2007, and four employees with chemical burns in 2006. These four employees were involved in a single incident that resulted in their burns. After our first visit in February 2010, one employee sought care at the emergency room for cough and chest pain after breathing in chemicals at work. He was treated with a bronchodilator and released with an inhaler to use if he became short of breath.

Air Sampling

Several compounds were detected on the VOC screening samples, including indene, ethyl acetate, toluene, benzene, naphthalene, methyl methacrylate, trimethyl benzene, xylene, and cumene. The latter three compounds are listed as components of Aromatic 100, which was used in the poly wash and tote wash departments. Many of these compounds were measured on the aromatic hydrocarbon samples. The PBZ concentrations of cumene, ethyl benzene, toluene, trimethyl benzene, and xylene are provided in Table 2. The MDCs and MQCs are also provided in Table 2. The MDCs and MQCs were calculated by dividing the analytical limits of detection and quantitation (mass units) by the minimum volume of air sampled. The MDCs and MQCs represent the smallest air concentrations that could have been detected (MDC) or quantified (MQC) for the volume of air sampled. Concentrations between the MDC and MQC are listed in Table 2 but are shown in parentheses to point out that there is more uncertainty associated with these values than with concentrations above the MQC. All exposures were below applicable OELs except one PBZ concentration of trimethyl benzene (150 mg/m^3) that was above the NIOSH REL and ACGIH TLV of 125 mg/m^3. This concentration was measured on March 22, 2010, in the PBZ of an employee in the tote wash department who wiped the exterior of the totes with Aromatic 100. On the following day, this employee's exposure was 83 mg/m^3.

RESULTS
(CONTINUED)

Indiana OSHA also reported than an employee in the tote wash department was overexposed to trimethyl benzene (330 mg/m³) on August 26, 2010 [IOSHA 2011].

The air sampling results for benzene and naphthalene are not provided in Table 2 because the concentrations of these compounds were near or below their MDCs. The MDC for benzene was 0.02 mg/m³ and the MDC for naphthalene was 0.03 mg/m³. These concentrations are well below applicable OELs.

Table 2. Work-shift PBZ concentrations of cumene, ethyl benzene, toluene, trimethyl benzene, and xylene

Dept.	Sample date	Job task	Cumene	Ethyl benzene	Toluene	Trimethyl benzenes	Xylene
Poly wash	3/22/2010	Remove labels*	0.043	0.028	(0.14)	13	0.18
		Wipe exterior with Dissolve II	0.1	0.053	(0.14)	28	0.31
		Wipe exterior with Aromatic 100	0.10	0.018	(0.096)	5.3	0.27
		Spray paint	0.14	0.024	0.44	6.2	0.36
	3/23/2010	Remove labels	0.039	0.026	ND	10	0.11
		Wipe exterior with Dissolve II	0.094	0.022	(0.062)	30	0.14
		Rebung	0.035	(0.0024)	ND	2.3	0.073
		Spray paint	0.080	0.016	1.3	3.8	0.19
Regrind	3/22/2010	Empty and vacuum*	0.031	0.082	(0.072)	5.3	0.46
	3/23/2010	Empty and vacuum	0.022	0.019	(0.046)	4.1	0.12
Tote wash	3/22/2010	Remove labels*	0.99	0.032	ND	45	1.8
		Wipe exterior with Aromatic 100	3.6	0.1	ND	150	6.6
	3/23/2010	Remove labels	0.58	0.016	ND	30	0.99
		Wipe exterior with Aromatic 100*	1.8	0.054	ND	83	3.4
MDC			0.003	0.003	0.07	0.01	0.007
MQC			0.015	0.015	0.22	0.044	0.029

*Samples collected over 6.5 hours or less. All other samples were collected over 7.5 hours or more.

The PBZ concentrations of sodium hydroxide were all ND (below the MDC of 0.04 mg/m^3). These air samples were collected in the PBZs of the employees who loaded and unloaded drums from the automatic caustic wash system in the poly wash department. Because the MDC is well below the NIOSH REL and ACGIH ceiling limit of 2 mg/m^3, we can be certain that these employees were not overexposed to sodium hydroxide during this evaluation.

Noise Monitoring

Table 3 summarizes personal noise exposure measurements by department and job task. All personal noise exposure measurements exceeded the NIOSH REL and the OSHA AL of 85 dBA for an 8-hour work shift. Additionally, noise exposures for employees loading drums, wiping the exterior of drums with Dissolve II, spraying drums and totes with pressurized water, emptying and vacuuming drums, and removing labels from totes exceeded the OSHA PEL of 90 dBA. Of particular note was that employees using pressure sprayers in the poly wash and tote wash departments had TWA noise exposures above 100 dBA, a noise exposure level at which NIOSH recommends the use of dual hearing protection (i.e., the combination of earplugs and earmuffs). A few employees wore dual protection; however, employees using pressure sprayers only wore single protection (foam insert earplugs). We noticed that several employees in the plant did not properly insert their disposable foam earplugs deep enough into the ear canal.

Sound level and one-third octave band noise measurements were taken at the pressure washing stations in the tote wash and poly wash departments. Overall sound levels for both were approximately 104 dB. For the drum pressure washer, high frequency noise from approximately 4,000 to 20,000 Hz was predominant. The tote pressure washer also had substantial noise in frequencies from 10,000 to 20,000 Hz. However, the tote pressure washer also had peaks at low frequencies of 80 Hz and to a somewhat lesser extent at 160 Hz. Octave band measurement results are shown in Figure 4.

Octave band measurements in the audiometric test booth (not shown) indicated that noise levels in the booth were below the maximum allowable levels specified by OSHA in Table D1 of the noise standard [29 CFR 1910.95].

RESULTS
(CONTINUED)

Table 3. Summary of personal work-shift TWA noise exposure measurements

Department	Job task	No. of samples	NIOSH REL (dBA)	OSHA AL (dBA)	OSHA PEL (dBA)
Indoor loading	Loading drums	4	88.8 – 98.0	86.5 – 96.6	81.3 – 96.3
Poly wash	Rebung	2	88.9 – 89.7	88.2 – 89.2	83.3 – 84.8
Poly wash	Spray paint	2	87.5 – 89.1	86.5 – 88.2	78.9 – 83.9
Poly wash	Wipe exterior with Dissolve II	2	94.8 – 96.0	93.7 – 94.5	92.9 – 94.2
Poly wash	Remove labels	2	90.9 – 91.3	90.2 – 90.5	87.2 – 88.1
Poly wash	Pressure wash drums	2	104.3 – 104.9	102.3 – 102.9	102.0 – 102.7
Regrind	Empty and vacuum drums	2	92 – 92.6	91.1 – 91.9	89.8 – 90.9
Regrind	Operate grinder	3	90.2 – 91.7	88.7 – 90.0	86.0 – 87.6
Regrind	Shredder	1	92.3	89.4	86.9
Tote wash	Remove labels	1	93.2	92.4	91.4
Tote wash	Pressure wash totes	2	98.4 – 102.1	97.1 – 100.3	96.9 – 100.2
Tote wash	Revalve	2	90.8 – 92.8	89.9 – 91.5	86.1 – 89.3
Noise Exposure Limits			85.0	85.0	90.0

Other Observations

All employees were required to wear safety glasses, hard hats, and steel-toed boots. PVC gloves with a cotton lining were provided to employees. Employees reported changing the gloves two times per week. An employee in the poly wash department was not wearing safety glasses and had cut off his glove cuffs so they no longer covered his wrists. This employee said he cut off the glove cuffs to make them more comfortable. Sleeve covers were available, but most employees did not wear them. Some employees did not store their gloves properly between uses. We observed gloves on the floor, on top of chemical drums, and on top of a plunger of solvent. Although the company provided PPE, no written PPE hazard assessment and documentation of employee training had been completed as required by OSHA [29 CFR 1910.132].

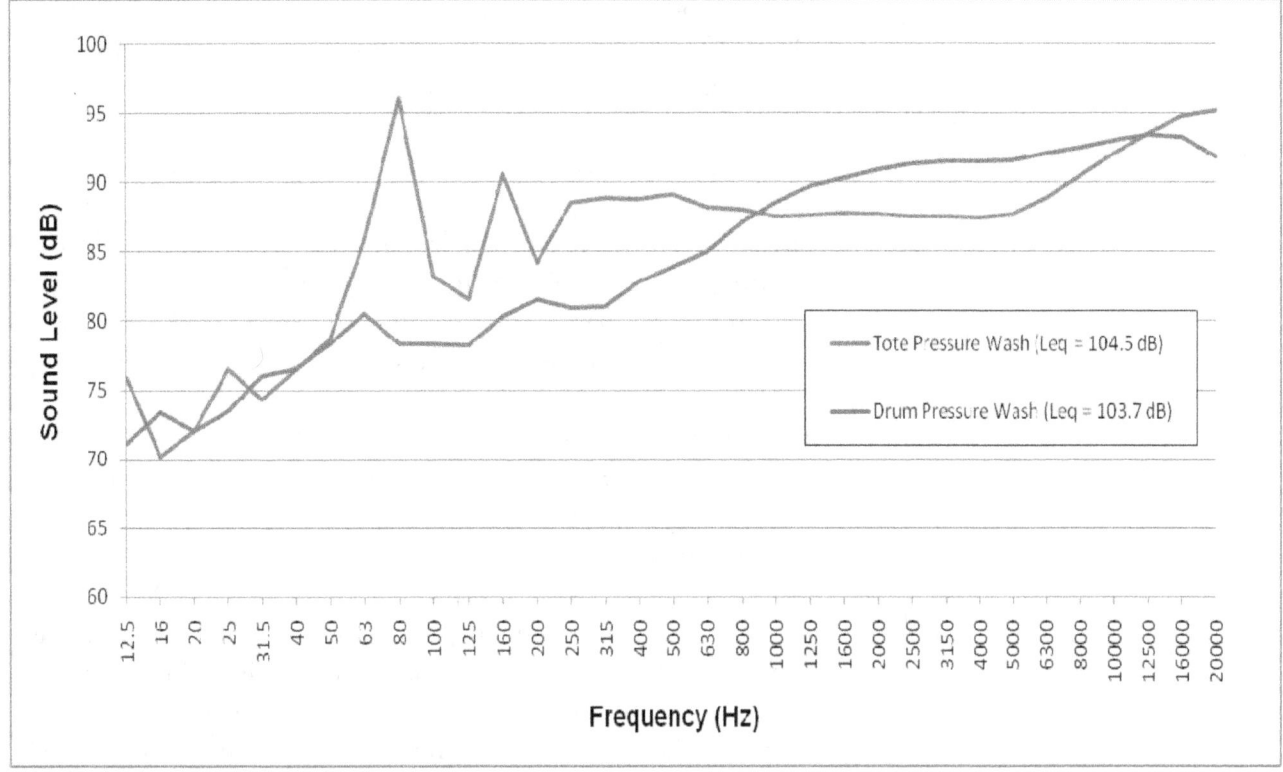

Figure 4. Octave band analysis for the tote pressure wash and drum pressure wash.

Half-mask N95 filtering facepiece respirators (model 8210, 3M, St. Paul, Minnesota) were available to employees for voluntary use. However, we observed employees who were improperly wearing and maintaining these respirators. Some employees believed that these respirators protected them against vapors and gases, but these respirators are only effective against particles.

Use of hearing protection was required in all production areas of the plant unless an employee intended to be in the plant for less than 20 minutes. However, hearing protection was required in the regrind department at all times. The company provided Howard Leight Sperian (San Diego, California) Max Lite foam insert hearing protectors with a noise reduction rating of 30 dB. Some employees were also provided with Howard Leight Model L2H earmuffs (noise reduction rating of 25 dB), which attached to their hardhats.

The company provided audiometric testing for all production employees. Previously, audiometric testing was conducted during the work shift in an empty house across the street from the plant. Personnel from the company's corporate office performed audiometric tests. We were told that future audiometric testing will be conducted by the safety director using a Beltone (Glenview, Illinois) Model 119 audiometer. The audiometric test booth is located in the warehouse building.

The electrical outlets in the poly wash department (near the automatic caustic wash machine) did not contain ground fault circuit interrupters. Additionally, the metal of electrical outlets and control panels was being corroded because of humidity and caustic mist in the area. This corrosion could present an electrical hazard because of the high moisture levels in this area.

Forklift drivers did not always wear seat belts and did not consistently use their horns prior to turning corners from one aisle to another, behavior that increases the risk of injury to forklift drivers and other employees.

The eyewash station in the regrind department had no protective covers over the nozzles, which could lead to debris blocking the flow of water. We observed unbalanced water spray from the nozzles at the eyewash station in the poly wash department by the hydraulic pump and at other eyewash stations in the plant.

Two open vats containing rinse water (approximately 3 feet in height) were not labeled. We also found unlabeled containers of Aromatic 100 and Dissolve II, most likely because the solvent had removed the labels. The wall fan in the tote wash department where an employee wiped the outside of the totes with Aromatic 100 was not operational during our visit.

Management at the plant held monthly "toolbox" meetings. These meetings covered a variety of topics, including safety issues, and were attended by all employees. However, the plant had no employee-management health and safety committee that met regularly to discuss health and safety concerns.

Chemical Exposures

Breathing and skin contact are important routes of exposure to organic solvents, or VOCs, in the workplace. Almost all organic solvents cause skin irritation because they remove fat from the skin. Organic solvents may also irritate the respiratory system. This irritation is usually restricted to the upper airways, mucous membranes, and eyes, and it generally resolves quickly without long-term effects. In addition, almost all volatile, fat-soluble organic solvents can cause acute nonspecific central nervous system depression. The symptoms of significant acute solvent exposure are similar to those from drinking too many alcoholic beverages, including headache, nausea and vomiting, dizziness, slurred speech, impaired balance, disorientation, and confusion. These symptoms go away quickly when exposure stops. Although most employees reported no symptoms, those who did reported eye and respiratory irritation, which are consistent with solvent exposure. Acids and caustics are also irritants.

The VOC air sampling results revealed the presence of many different compounds in employees' PBZs. Some of these compounds (cumene, xylene, and trimethyl benzene) were listed in the MSDS for Aromatic 100. The other VOCs we detected in air could have been from the volatilization of Dissolve II or residual chemicals in the drums. It is important to note that the VOC air samples are not able to measure all chemicals in the air. Therefore, other hazardous chemicals could have been present in the air during our evaluation. This would include inorganic decomposition products (e.g., carbon monoxide, chlorine, hydrogen cyanide, etc.) from the mixing of incompatible chemicals.

Except for trimethyl benzene, the PBZ concentrations of the aromatic hydrocarbons and sodium hydroxide were well below applicable OELs. The source of trimethyl benzene for the overexposed employee was most likely the Aromatic 100 that was used liberally to clean the exterior of the totes. The wall fan near the employee performing this activity was not operating during our visit so less general dilution ventilation was in the area, which could allow vapors to accumulate in his PBZ. This employee performed the same job task on the following day and was exposed to 83 mg/m^3 of trimethyl benzene, which is two thirds of the OEL. Thus, his overexposure to trimethyl benzene is not likely to be an unusual occurrence. The employee in the poly wash department who scrubbed the exterior of the drums with Dissolve II was exposed to around 30 mg/m^3 of trimethyl benzene on both sample days. While these exposures are less than a quarter of the OELs, they suggest that Dissolve II may be another source of trimethyl benzene. Moreover, higher trimethyl benzene exposures could be expected in the warmer summer months because the plant does not have air conditioning, and the volatility of chemicals increases with rising temperatures. For example, Indiana OSHA measured PBZ concentrations of trimethyl benzene in the tote wash department during the summer (August 2010) that were more than twice what we measured in the same area in the spring (March 2010) [IOSHA 2011]. Also, the chemicals in the drums vary over time, which could lead to a different mixture and concentration of chemicals in the air.

Employees at the plant have the potential for dermal exposures. Employees who handle Dissolve II and Aromatic 100, in particular, could expose their hands to aromatic and petroleum-based hydrocarbons if they do not wear the proper type of gloves or change them frequently enough. Dipropylene glycol monomethyl ether, a component of Dissolve II, could also present a hazard to poorly protected skin. The PVC gloves worn by employees were changed two times per week. According to the Quick Selection Guide to Chemical Protective Clothing [Forsberg and Mansdorf 2007], cumene and xylene, both constituents of Aromatic 100, can penetrate PVC gloves in less than 1 hour. (PVC gloves were not evaluated against dipropylene glycol monomethyl ether.) Skin contact of cumene and xylene could potentially lead to skin problems, including contact dermatitis, or dermal absorption and systemic uptake of aromatic hydrocarbons [ILO 1989]. However, other than four cases of chemical burns in 2006, employees did not report having skin problems.

Noise Exposures

All monitored employees' TWA noise exposures exceeded the NIOSH REL and the OSHA AL of 85 dBA. Employees using pressure sprayers in the poly wash and tote wash departments had TWA noise exposures above 100 dBA. All of these employees should remain in the hearing conservation program and be required to wear hearing protection. Until noise exposures are reduced to below 100 dBA, employees pressure washing drums and totes should be required to wear earplugs and earmuffs. Because we observed several employees who did not insert hearing protectors deeply enough into their ear canal, all employees should be retrained on how to properly insert earplugs. Improperly worn earplugs do not provide enough protection from noise. Supervisors should be responsible for observing hearing protection use and should help ensure the hearing protection is worn correctly.

The highest noise levels in the plant occur during pressure washing of drums or totes. Sound levels over 100 dBA were measured during these tasks and were high enough to affect noise exposures in adjacent work areas. For example, noise levels in the tote valve installer station about 25 feet from the pressure wash station were approximately 86 dBA when the pressure washer was not operating, but increased to 95 dBA when the pressure washer was operating. Because much of the noise generated by the pressure wash is high frequency, partial enclosures or barrier walls may be effective in reducing noise levels in adjacent areas. However, an enclosure would not reduce exposure for employees while pressure washing. Alternatively, an enclosed and automated pressure washing system could be designed and installed to wash the exterior of drums and totes. This system would protect those doing the job and those in adjacent areas.

We noted that several employee audiograms showed year-to-year variation in HTLs. While a variation of 5 to 10 dB in HTL from one audiogram to the next is common, an improvement in HTL greater than 10 dB is not a typical pattern. There may be several reasons for this variability. Because audiograms were conducted during the work shift, some employees may have had a TTS at the time of an audiogram, but did not have a TTS for the next audiogram. A TTS could occur because employees were exposed to noise but did not wear hearing protection before the audiogram or their hearing protection was not properly worn, allowing for substantial noise exposure. It is also possible that there was excessive background noise during the employee's audiometric test, which may have resulted in an artificially high HTL for that particular test. Prior to 2009, an empty house across the street was used for audiometric testing.

Personal Protective Equipment Hazard Assessment

OSHA requires all employers to complete a comprehensive assessment of their workplaces to determine if hazards are present, or likely to be present, that would require the use of PPE such as safety glasses, protective gloves, safety shoes, or other PPE. Lack of appropriate PPE may result in injuries, including eye injuries caused

DISCUSSION
(CONTINUED)

by projected debris or chemical splashes, burns or skin injuries from chemical splashes, skin absorption of hazardous chemical agents, head or foot injuries from falling objects, lacerations from sharp objects or edges, and trauma from falls. Employees must also be trained to know when PPE must be used, what type of PPE is required, how to properly adjust and wear the PPE, what are the limitations of the PPE (e.g., what it will not protect them against), how to properly take care of the PPE, or in the case of disposable PPE, how to know when it is time to dispose of it. OSHA requires the employer to document in writing that the PPE hazard assessment and employee training have been completed.

CONCLUSIONS

We measured an overexposure to trimethyl benzene in the air and found that skin exposure to aromatic and petroleum-based hydrocarbons may occur if proper gloves are not worn or changed frequently. Some employees reported symptoms that were consistent with exposures from airborne exposures to solvents. Most employees were exposed to high noise levels that exceeded NIOSH and OSHA exposure limits. Some employees were exposed to noise levels greater than 100 dBA, an exposure level for which NIOSH recommends wearing wear earplugs and earmuffs to protect employee hearing.

RECOMMENDATIONS

On the basis of our findings, we recommend the actions listed below to create a more healthful workplace. We encourage the plant to use a labor-management health and safety committee or working group to discuss the recommendations in this report and develop an action plan. Those involved in the work can best set priorities and assess the feasibility of our recommendations for the specific situation at the plant. Our recommendations are based on the hierarchy of controls approach (Appendix B: Occupational Exposure Limits and Health Effects). This approach groups actions by their likely effectiveness in reducing or removing hazards. In most cases, the preferred approach is to eliminate hazardous materials or processes and install engineering controls to reduce exposure or shield employees. Until such controls are in place, or if they are not effective or feasible, administrative measures and/or personal protective equipment may be needed.

Elimination and Substitution

Elimination or substitution of a toxic/hazardous process material is a highly effective means for reducing hazards. Incorporating this strategy into the design or development phase of a project, commonly referred to as "prevention through design" is most effective because it reduces the need for additional controls in the future.

1. Substitute Aromatic 100 with a less hazardous solvent for cleaning the outside of totes and drums. Aromatic 100 was the primary source for the trimethyl benzene that led to an employee being overexposed in the tote wash department.

Engineering Controls

Engineering controls reduce exposures to employees by removing the hazard from the process or placing a barrier between the hazard and the employee. Engineering controls are very effective at protecting employees without placing primary responsibility of implementation on the employee.

1. Add local exhaust ventilation to the work areas where drums and totes are emptied and cleaned. Although we identified only an overexposure to trimethyl benzene, other hazardous chemicals in the drums could volatilize into the air. A downdraft or crossdraft exhaust ventilation system would remove potentially hazardous vapors and gases at the floor level before they are able to reach the PBZs of the employees.

2. Install an exhaust hood over the drums used to collect residual waste emptied from the totes. An exhaust hood would remove potentially hazardous chemicals that evaporate from the drums.

3. Partially enclose or install barrier walls in the noisiest areas of the plant (i.e., where drums and totes are pressure washed) to reduce noise levels in adjacent work areas. Alternatively, an enclosed and automated pressure washing system could be designed and installed to wash the exterior of drums and totes.

4. Install electrical outlets containing ground fault circuit interrupters in the poly wash department (near the automatic caustic wash machine) to prevent electrical hazards.

5. Add protective covers to the nozzles of eyewash stations and ensure an evenly distributed flow of water between nozzles for all eyewash stations. In addition, inspect and test the eyewash stations monthly to ensure they work properly and document that they have been tested.

Administrative Controls

Administrative controls are management-dictated work practices, policies, and programs to reduce or prevent exposures to workplace hazards. The effectiveness of administrative controls is dependent on management commitment and employee acceptance. Regular monitoring and reinforcement are necessary to ensure that control policies and procedures are not circumvented in the name of convenience or production.

1. Follow the recommendations from Indiana OSHA to segregate the cleaning of drums and totes according to the types of chemicals they contain to prevent exothermic reactions or the release of hazardous decomposition products. This would also facilitate the proper neutralization, disposal, and hazard communication requirements of the collected materials [IOSHA 2011].

2. Add labels to the unlabeled vats containing rinse water in the poly wash department. This informs employees and emergency personnel about the contents of the vats.

3. Add laminated tags to the unlabeled containers of Aromatic 100 and Dissolve II to identify the contents and provide health hazard warning information. This information helps protect employees and prevent misuse of the products. The solvent should not cause the tags to fall off.

4. Start an employee-management health and safety committee that meets regularly to discuss health and safety concerns.

Personal Protective Equipment

PPE is the least effective means for controlling employee exposures. Proper use of PPE requires a comprehensive program, and calls for a high level of employee involvement and commitment to be effective. The use of PPE requires the choice of the appropriate equipment to reduce the hazard and the development of supporting programs such as training, change-out schedules,

RECOMMENDATIONS
(CONTINUED)

and medical assessment if needed. PPE should not be relied upon as the sole method for limiting employee exposures. Rather, PPE should be used until engineering and administrative controls can be demonstrated to be effective in limiting exposures to acceptable levels.

1. Conduct a comprehensive hazard assessment to facilitate the selection of PPE as required by OSHA [29 CFR 1910.132]. Compliance assistance and guidelines for hazard assessment and PPE selection are provided in 29 CFR 1910 Subpart I Appendix B. OSHA eTools, available at http://www.osha.gov/dts/osta/oshasoft/, provides additional resources for PPE selection. Indiana OSHA has a free consultation program called *INSafe*, available at http://www.in.gov/dol/2379.htm that could provide assistance with the PPE hazard assessment. Document that the PPE hazard assessment and employee training have been completed.

2. Retrain employees on how to properly wear and maintain PPE, including hearing protection, gloves, sleeve covers, and safety glasses. Supervisors should be responsible for observing and ensuring the correct use of PPE.

3. Choose new gloves for employees who handle Aromatic 100 and Dissolve II. The PVC gloves currently used are not protective against aromatic hydrocarbons (breakthrough of cumene and xylene in less than 1 hour is possible). The *Quick Selection Guide to Chemical Protective Clothing* [Forsberg and Mansdorf 2007] provides information that can be used in selecting more protective gloves and change-out schedules. On the basis of protection and cost of gloves, we recommend using thick (>10 millimeter) nitrile gloves and, at a minimum, changing out these gloves midway through the workday (after lunch). Gloves should also be rinsed and stored properly (away from chemicals) between uses.

4. Require employees who pressure wash drums and totes to wear earplugs and earmuffs until their TWA noise exposures are reduced to below 100 dBA.

5. Stop using N95 filtering facepiece respirators. These respirators are intended for particle exposures. During our evaluations, we did not observe particle exposures. If particle exposures are occurring and the PBZ concentrations are below applicable OELs, then these respirators can be provided for voluntary

RECOMMENDATIONS (CONTINUED)

use. However, employees should be told that these respirators do not provide protection against vapors or gases. In addition, employees should be trained on the proper wear and maintenance of such respirators. Although a written respiratory protection program is not mandatory for voluntary use of respirators with this level of protection, OSHA requires that employees be provided a copy of Appendix D, "Information for Employees Using Respirators When Not Required Under the Standard," of the OSHA Respiratory Protection Standard [29 CFR 1910.134].

REFERENCES

ACGIH [2010]. Threshold limit values for chemical substances and physical agents and biological exposure indices. Cincinnati, OH: American Conference of Governmental Industrial Hygienists.

CFR. Code of Federal Regulations. Washington, DC: U.S. Government Printing Office, Office of the Federal Register.

Forsberg K, Mansdorf SZ [2007]. Quick Selection Guide to Chemical Protective Clothing Fifth Edition. Hoboken, NJ: Wiley-Interscience.

ILO [1989]. Hydrocarbons, aromatic. In: Stellman JM, ed. International Labour Office encyclopaedia. 4th ed. Geneva, Switzerland: International Labour Office (ILO).

IOSHA [2011]. Safety order and notification of penalty. Indianapolis, IN: Indiana Department of Labor, Indiana Occupational Safety and Health Administration (IOSHA) Publication No. 313128068. [http://www.osha.gov/pls/imis/establishment.html]. Date accessed: April 2011.

NIOSH [2005]. NIOSH pocket guide to chemical hazards. Barsen ME, ed. Cincinnati, OH: U.S. Department of Health and Human Services, Centers for Disease Control and Prevention, National Institute for Occupational Safety and Health (NIOSH) Publication No. 2005-149.

Air Sampling for Volatile Organic Compounds

Thermal desorption tubes were used to sample air in the PBZs of the employees. The thermal desorption tubes contained three beds of sorbent material: (1) 90 mg of Carbopack™ Y, (2) 115 mg of Carbopack B, and (3) 150 mg of Carboxen™. Calibrated Aircheck 2000 pumps (SKC Incorporated, Eighty Four, Pennsylvania) were used for drawing airflows of 50 cc/min through the sampling media. The samples were qualitatively analyzed for various VOCs according to NIOSH Method 2549 [NIOSH 2011].

Air Sampling for Aromatic Hydrocarbons

Charcoal tubes (100 mg/50 mg) were used to sample air in the PBZs of the employees. Calibrated SKC Aircheck 2000 pumps pulled 200 cc/min of air through the sampling media. The samples were analyzed for cumene, ethylbenzene, naphthalene, toluene, trimethyl benzene, xylene, and benzene according to NIOSH Method 1501 [NIOSH 2011].

Noise Sampling

Larson-Davis (Provo, Utah) Spark® 705P noise dosimeters were worn by employees while they performed their daily activities. The noise dosimeters were attached to the wearers' belts, and small remote microphones were fastened to the wearers' shirts at a point midway between the ear and the outside of the shoulder. Windscreens provided by the dosimeter manufacturer were placed over the microphones during measurements to reduce or eliminate artifact noise, which can occur if objects bump against an unprotected microphone. The dosimeters were set up to collect data using different settings so that we could directly compare the noise measurement results with the three different noise exposure limits referenced in this HHE, the OSHA PEL and AL, and the NIOSH REL. OSHA uses a 90-dBA criterion and a 5-dB exchange rate. The difference between the OSHA PEL and AL is the threshold level used for each. The PEL has a 90-dBA threshold, and the AL has an 80-dBA threshold. NIOSH has an 85-dBA criterion and uses a 80-dBA threshold. During noise dosimetry measurements, noise levels below the threshold level are not integrated by the dosimeter for accumulation of dose and calculation of TWA noise level.

The dosimeters averaged noise levels every second during monitoring. At the end of the sampling period, the dosimeters were removed and paused to stop data collection. The noise measurement information stored in the dosimeters was downloaded to a personal computer for interpretation with Larson Davis Blaze® computer software. The dosimeters were calibrated before and after the measurement periods according to the manufacturer's instructions.

Area noise levels and octave band frequency spectrum analysis (measurement of noise in different frequencies) were measured with System 824 SLM and real-time frequency analyzers (Larson-Davis, Provo, Utah). The SLMs were equipped with 0.5-inch random incidence Type 1 electret microphones and the instruments measured noise levels between 16 and 157 dBA. The SLMs were calibrated before and after the measurement periods according to the manufacturer's instructions. SLMs were either handheld or mounted on a tripod at a height of approximately 5 feet.

References

NIOSH [2011]. NIOSH manual of analytical methods. 4th ed. Schlecht PC, O'Connor PF, eds. Cincinnati, OH: U.S. Department of Health and Human Services, Centers for Disease Control and Prevention, National Institute for Occupational Safety and Health, DHHS (NIOSH) Publication No. 94-113 (August 1994); 1st Supplement Publication 96-135, 2nd Supplement Publication 98-119, 3rd Supplement Publication 2003-154. [http://www.cdc.gov/niosh/docs/2003-154/]. Date accessed: April 2011.

Appendix B: Occupational Exposure Limits and Health Effects

In evaluating the hazards posed by workplace exposures, NIOSH investigators use both mandatory (legally enforceable) and recommended OELs for chemical, physical, and biological agents as a guide for making recommendations. OELs have been developed by federal agencies and safety and health organizations to prevent the occurrence of adverse health effects from workplace exposures. Generally, OELs suggest levels of exposure that most employees may be exposed to for up to 10 hours per day, 40 hours per week, for a working lifetime, without experiencing adverse health effects. However, not all employees will be protected from adverse health effects even if their exposures are maintained below these levels. A small percentage may experience adverse health effects because of individual susceptibility, a preexisting medical condition, and/or a hypersensitivity (allergy). In addition, some hazardous substances may act in combination with other workplace exposures, the general environment, or with medications or personal habits of the employee to produce adverse health effects even if the occupational exposures are controlled at the level set by the exposure limit. Also, some substances can be absorbed by direct contact with the skin and mucous membranes in addition to being inhaled, which contributes to the individual's overall exposure.

Most OELs are expressed as a TWA exposure. A TWA refers to the average exposure during a normal 8- to 10-hour workday. Some chemical substances and physical agents have recommended STEL or ceiling values where adverse health effects are caused by exposures over a short period. Unless otherwise noted, the STEL is a 15-minute TWA exposure that should not be exceeded at any time during a workday, and the ceiling limit is an exposure that should not be exceeded at any time.

In the United States, OELs have been established by federal agencies, professional organizations, state and local governments, and other entities. Some OELs are legally enforceable limits, while others are recommendations. The U.S. Department of Labor OSHA PELs (29 CFR 1910 [general industry]; 29 CFR 1926 [construction industry]; and 29 CFR 1917 [maritime industry]) are legal limits enforceable in workplaces covered under the Occupational Safety and Health Act of 1970. NIOSH RELs are recommendations based on a critical review of the scientific and technical information available on a given hazard and the adequacy of methods to identify and control the hazard. NIOSH RELs can be found in the *NIOSH Pocket Guide to Chemical Hazards* [NIOSH 2005]. NIOSH also recommends different types of risk management practices (e.g., engineering controls, safe work practices, employee education/training, personal protective equipment, and exposure and medical monitoring) to minimize the risk of exposure and adverse health effects from these hazards. Other OELs that are commonly used and cited in the United States include the TLVs recommended by ACGIH, a professional organization, and the WEELs recommended by the American Industrial Hygiene Association, another professional organization. The TLVs and WEELs are developed by committee members of these associations from a review of the published, peer-reviewed literature. They are not consensus standards. ACGIH TLVs are considered voluntary exposure guidelines for use by industrial hygienists and others trained in this discipline "to assist in the control of health hazards" [ACGIH 2010]. WEELs have been established for some chemicals "when no other legal or authoritative limits exist" [AIHA 2010].

Outside the United States, OELs have been established by various agencies and organizations and include both legal and recommended limits. The Institut für Arbeitsschutz der Deutschen Gesetzlichen Unfallversicherung (IFA, Institute for Occupational Safety and Health of the German Social Accident Insurance) maintains a database of international OELs from European Union member states, Canada (Québec), Japan, Switzerland, and the United States. The database, available at http://www.dguv.de/ifa/en/gestis/limit_values/index.jsp, contains international limits for over 1,500 hazardous substances and is updated periodically.

Employers should understand that not all hazardous chemicals have specific OSHA PELs, and for some agents the legally enforceable and recommended limits may not reflect current health-based information. However, an employer is still required by OSHA to protect its employees from hazards even in the absence of a specific OSHA PEL. OSHA requires an employer to furnish employees a place of employment free from recognized hazards that cause or are likely to cause death or serious physical harm [Occupational Safety and Health Act of 1970 (Public Law 91–596, sec. 5(a)(1))]. Thus, NIOSH investigators encourage employers to make use of other OELs when making risk assessments and risk management decisions to best protect the health of their employees. NIOSH investigators also encourage the use of the traditional hierarchy of controls approach to eliminate or minimize identified workplace hazards. This includes, in order of preference, the use of (1) substitution or elimination of the hazardous agent, (2) engineering controls (e.g., local exhaust ventilation, process enclosure, dilution ventilation), (3) administrative controls (e.g., limiting time of exposure, employee training, work practice changes, medical surveillance), and (4) personal protective equipment (e.g., respiratory protection, gloves, eye protection, hearing protection). Control banding, a qualitative risk assessment and risk management tool, is a complementary approach to protecting employee health that focuses resources on exposure controls by describing how a risk needs to be managed. Information on control banding is available at http://www.cdc.gov/niosh/topics/ctrlbanding/. This approach can be applied in situations where OELs have not been established or can be used to supplement the OELs, when available.

A PBZ concentration of trimethyl benzene and several personal noise exposures exceeded applicable OELs. The PBZ concentrations of the other compounds we sampled were well below their applicable OELs. Therefore, we only discuss the potential health effects from exposure to trimethyl benzene and noise. However, health effect information for the other compounds is available at http://www.cdc.gov/niosh/ipcs/nicstart.html.

Trimethyl Benzene

Short-term exposures to trimethyl benzene can cause irritation to the eyes, skin, and respiratory tract. Long-term exposures can defat the skin, and cause chronic bronchitis and adverse effects on the blood and central nervous systems [IPCS 2002]. The NIOSH REL and ACGIH TLV for trimethyl benzene pertains to the three isomers (1,3,5-trimethyl benzene, 1,2,4-trimethyl benzene, and 1,2,3-trimethyl benzene). The NIOSH REL for trimethyl benzene was adopted from the OSHA PEL of 125 mg/m^3 that was established for the three isomers of trimethyl benzene in 1989, but vacated by the 11th Circuit Court of Appeals in 1992 [NIOSH 2005]. Nevertheless, OSHA can use the 1989 PEL (current NIOSH REL) for trimethyl benzene to justify violations of the "general duty clause" as contained in Section 5(a) (1) of the Occupational Safety and Health Act [29 USC 1900]. The ACGIH TLV is intended to minimize changes to the central nervous system, asthmatic bronchitis, and blood dyscrasias (an abnormal blood condition) [ACGIH 2001]. The latter health effect could be due to the contamination of trimethyl benzene with benzene. For this reason it is important to measure benzene when products containing trimethyl benzene are being used [ACGIH 2001].

Noise

Noise-induced hearing loss is an irreversible, sensorineural condition that progresses with exposure. Although hearing ability declines with age (presbycusis), noise exposure produces more hearing loss than that resulting from aging alone. This noise-induced hearing loss is caused by damage to nerve cells of the inner ear (cochlea) and, unlike some conductive hearing disorders, cannot be treated medically [Berger et al. 2003]. In most cases, noise-induced hearing loss develops slowly and usually occurs before it is noticed. Hearing loss is often severe enough to permanently affect a person's ability to hear and understand speech. For example, people with hearing loss may not be able to distinguish words such as "fish" from "fist." [Suter 1978].

The dBA is the preferred unit for measuring sound levels to assess employee noise exposures. The dBA noise scale is weighted to approximate the sensory response of human ears to sound frequencies near the hearing threshold. Because the dBA scale is logarithmic, increases of 3 dBA, 10 dBA, and 20 dBA represent a doubling, tenfold increase, and hundredfold increase of sound energy, respectively. Noise exposures expressed in dBA cannot be averaged by taking the arithmetic mean.

The OSHA noise standard [29 CFR 1910.95] specifies a PEL of 90 dBA, as an 8-hour TWA. The OSHA PEL is calculated using a 5-dB exchange rate. This means that a person may be exposed to noise levels of 95 dBA for no more than 4 hours, 100 dBA for 2 hours, 105 dBA for 1 hour, etc. Conversely, up to 16 hours exposure to 85 dBA is allowed by this exchange rate. An employee's daily noise dose, based on the duration and intensity of noise exposure, can be calculated according to the formula

$$\text{Dose} = 100 \times (C_1/T_1 + C_2/T_2 + ... + C_n/T_n),$$

where C_n indicates the total time of exposure at a specific noise level and T_n indicates the reference duration for that level as given in Table G-16a of the OSHA noise regulation. Doses greater than 100% are in excess of the OSHA PEL.

When noise exposures exceed the PEL of 90 dBA, OSHA requires that employees wear hearing protection, and that an employer implement feasible engineering or administrative controls to reduce noise exposures. The OSHA noise standard also requires an employer to implement a hearing conservation program when 8-hour TWA noise exposures exceed the AL of 85 dBA. The program must include noise monitoring, employee notification, observation, audiometric testing, hearing protectors, training, and record keeping.

NIOSH [NIOSH 1998] and ACGIH [ACGIH 2010] recommend an exposure limit of 85 dBA, as an 8-hour TWA. A more conservative 3-dB exchange rate is used in calculating these exposure limits. Using NIOSH criteria, an employee can be exposed to 85 dBA for 8 hours, but to no more than 88 dBA for 4 hours, 91 dBA for 2 hours, 94 dBA for 1 hour, etc. Twelve-hour exposures have to be 83.2 dBA or less according to the NIOSH REL.

Audiometric evaluations of employees' hearing thresholds must be conducted in quiet locations, preferably in a sound-attenuating booth, by presenting pure tones of varying frequencies at threshold levels (i.e., the level of a sound that the person can just barely hear). Zero dB HTL represents the hearing level of an average, young individual with good hearing. The OSHA hearing conservation standard requires hearing thresholds to be measured at test frequencies of 500, 1000, 2000, 3000, 4000, and 6000 Hz. Individual employee's annual audiograms are compared to their baseline audiogram to determine if an STS has occurred. OSHA states that an STS has occurred if the average threshold values at 2000, 3000, and 4000 Hz have increased by 10 dB or more in either ear when comparing the annual audiogram to the baseline audiogram [29 CFR 1910.95]. The NIOSH-recommended hearing threshold shift criterion is a 15-dB shift at any frequency in either ear from 500–6000 Hz measured twice in succession [NIOSH 1998]. Both of these hearing threshold shift criteria require at least two audiometric tests.

References

ACGIH [2001]. Trimethyl benzene, isomers. In: Documentation of the threshold limit values and biological exposure indices. Cincinnati, OH: American Conference of Governmental Industrial Hygienists.

ACGIH [2010]. Threshold limit values for chemical substances and physical agents and biological exposure indices. Cincinnati, OH: Arican Conference of Governmental Industrial Hygienists.

AIHA [2010]. AIHA 2010 Emergency response planning guidelines (ERPG) & workplace environmental exposure levels (WEEL) handbook. Fairfax, VA: American Industrial Hygiene Association.

Berger EH, Royster LH, Royster JD, Driscoll DP, Layne M, eds. [2003]. The noise manual. 5th rev. ed. Fairfax, VA: American Industrial Hygiene Association.

CFR. Code of Federal Regulations. Washington, DC: U.S. Government Printing Office, Office of the Federal Register.

IPCS (WHO/International Programme on Chemical Safety) [2002]. International Chemical Safety card: trimethyl benzene (mixed isomers). [http://www.cdc.gov/niosh/ipcsneng/neng1389.html]. Date accessed: April 2011.

NIOSH [1998]. Criteria for a recommended standard: Occupational noise exposure (revised criteria 1998). Cincinnati, OH: U.S. Department of Health and Human Services, Centers for Disease Control and Prevention, National Institute for Occupational Safety and Health, DHHS (NIOSH) Publication No. 98-126.

NIOSH [2005]. NIOSH pocket guide to chemical hazards. Barsen ME, ed. Cincinnati, OH: U.S. Department of Health and Human Services, Centers for Disease Control and Prevention, National Institute for Occupational Safety and Health (NIOSH) Publication No. 2005-149.

Suter AH [1978]. The ability of mildly-impaired individuals to discriminate speech in noise. Washington, DC: U.S. Environmental Protection Agency, Joint EPA/USAF study, EPA 550/9-78-100, AMRL-TR-78-4.

USC. United States Code. Washington, DC: U.S. Government Printing Office.

This page left intentionally blank

Acknowledgments and Availability of Report

The Hazard Evaluations and Technical Assistance Branch (HETAB) of the National Institute for Occupational Safety and Health (NIOSH) conducts field investigations of possible health hazards in the workplace. These investigations are conducted under the authority of Section 20(a)(6) of the Occupational Safety and Health Act of 1970, 29 U.S.C. 669(a)(6) which authorizes the Secretary of Health and Human Services, following a written request from any employer or authorized representative of employees, to determine whether any substance normally found in the place of employment has potentially toxic effects in such concentrations as used or found. HETAB also provides, upon request, technical and consultative assistance to federal, state, and local agencies; labor; industry; and other groups or individuals to control occupational health hazards and to prevent related trauma and disease.

The findings and conclusions in this report are those of the authors and do not necessarily represent the views of NIOSH. Mention of any company or product does not constitute endorsement by NIOSH. In addition, citations to websites external to NIOSH do not constitute NIOSH endorsement of the sponsoring organizations or their programs or products. Furthermore, NIOSH is not responsible for the content of these websites. All Web addresses referenced in this document were accessible as of the publication date.

This report was prepared by Kenneth W. Fent, Elena Page, and Scott E. Brueck of HETAB, Division of Surveillance, Hazard Evaluations and Field Studies. Industrial hygiene field assistance was provided by Greg Burr. Analytical support was provided by Ardith Grote. Health communication assistance was provided by Stefanie Evans. Editorial assistance was provided by Ellen Galloway. Desktop publishing was performed by Greg Hartle.

Copies of this report have been sent to employee and management representatives at the drum refurbishing plant, the Indian State Department of Health, the Indiana Occupational Safety and Health Administration, and the Occupational Safety and Health Administration Region 5 Office. This report is not copyrighted and may be freely reproduced. The report may be viewed and printed at http://www.cdc.gov/niosh/hhe/. Copies may be purchased from the National Technical Information Service at 5825 Port Royal Road, Springfield, Virginia 22161.

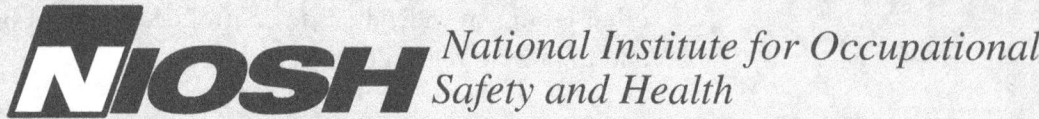

National Institute for Occupational Safety and Health

Delivering on the Nation's promise: Safety and health at work for all people through research and prevention.

To receive NIOSH documents or information about occupational safety and health topics, contact NIOSH at:

1-800-CDC-INFO (1-800-232-4636)

TTY: 1-888-232-6348

E-mail: cdcinfo@cdc.gov

or visit the NIOSH web site at: **www.cdc.gov/niosh.**

For a monthly update on news at NIOSH, subscribe to NIOSH eNews by visiting **www.cdc.gov/niosh/eNews.**

SAFER • HEALTHIER • PEOPLE™